THE "CAN" IN CANCER

published by

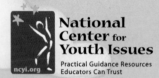
National Center for Youth Issues
Practical Guidance Resources
Educators Can Trust

ncyi.org

www.ncyi.org

To Nurse Twyla, with love.
–Julia

Disclaimer

This book is written to provide information about childhood cancer and should not be used as an alternative to receiving medical advice.
Every effort has been made to ensure that the information in this book is accurate at the time of publishing; however, there is no guarantee that the information will remain current over time. Always seek the advice of a trained professional.

Duplication and Copyright

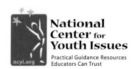

National Center for Youth Issues
Practical Guidance Resources
Educators Can Trust
ncyi.org

P.O. Box 22185 • Chattanooga, TN 37422-2185
423.899.5714 • 866.318.6294 • fax: 423.899.4547 • www.ncyi.org
ISBN: 978-1-937870-17-1
© 2013 National Center for Youth Issues, Chattanooga, TN
All rights reserved.

Written by: Julia Cook • Illustrations by: Allison Valentine
Design by: Phillip W. Rodgers • Contributing Editor: Beth Spencer Rabon
Published by National Center for Youth Issues
Softcover

Printed at Starkey Printing • Chattanooga, Tennessee, U.S.A. • July 2016

Forward

Having a child diagnosed with cancer is one of the most difficult crises that any parent will ever endure. It can be devastating to the family and overwhelming to all those who love the child.

Treatment for childhood cancer is often aggressive and can involve months to years of surgery, chemotherapy and radiation. 'Normal' daily life is transformed to a 'new normal' with the child spending extensive time in the hospital often feeling sick, tired and afraid. The child's life is filled with new limitations which can include missing school, not participating in sports and hobbies, and not playing with friends. Parents spend time away from work and siblings are often cared for by extended family members and friends. Families are often immobilized with the fear that life will never return to what it was prior to the child's diagnosis.

Julia Cook's *The "CAN" in CANCER* is a powerful book that teaches the child, the child's family and friends the importance of focusing on the things that "CAN" be achieved even when fighting cancer. By focusing on the things that "CAN" be accomplished instead of the things that "CAN'T," the child is able to find courage and hope from within, and share that courage and hope with others, so that they too can be inspired to find the "CAN" in their lives.

Ruth I. Hoffman, MPH
Executive Director
American Childhood Cancer Organization
www.acco.org

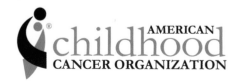

This book was made possible through the generosity of

Children's
HOSPITAL & MEDICAL CENTER
OMAHA

My name is Eli, and
I'm just a regular kid.

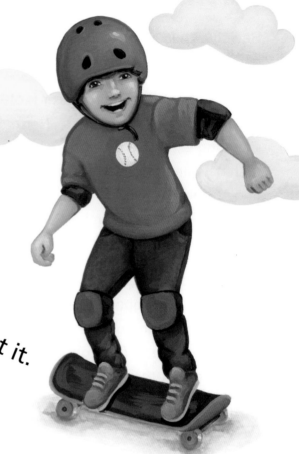

I like to skateboard, and I'm pretty good at it.

I don't like to read stories
that are boring.

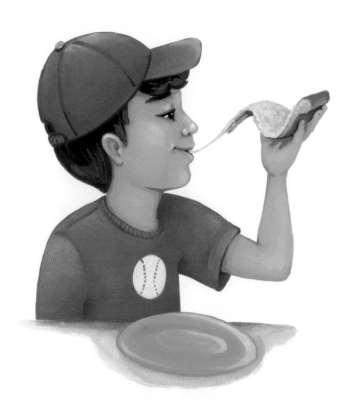

My favorite food is cheese pizza, but sometimes I eat hamburger pizza too.

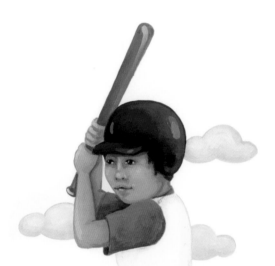

And, I LOVE, **LOVE**, **LOVE** to play baseball!

If I could play baseball every minute of every day of every week of every month for a whole year straight, I would be happy.

About a year ago, I started to get really, really tired all of the time.

I was too tired to skateboard.

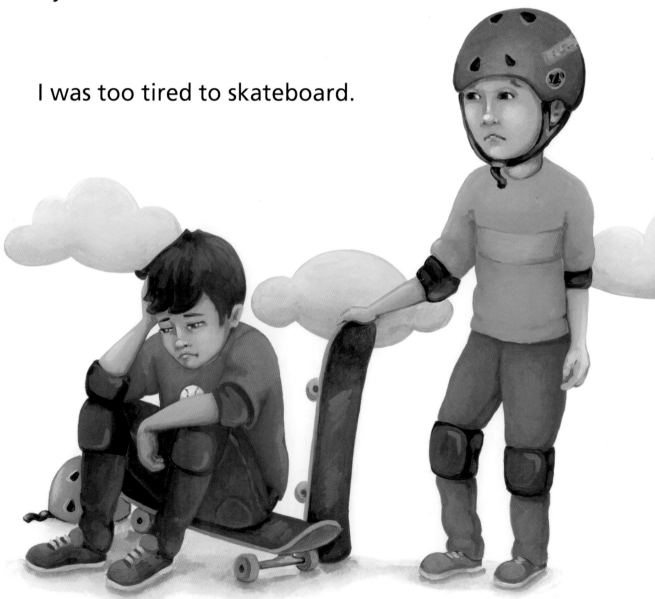

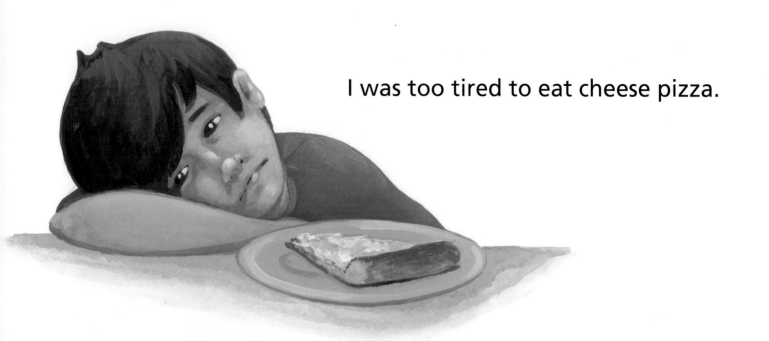

I was too tired to eat cheese pizza.

I was even too tired to play my baseball video games!

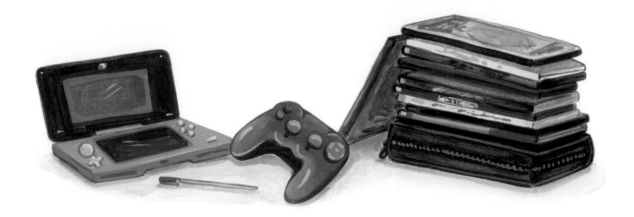

My mom started to worry about me,
so she took me to see the doctor.

That was a day I will NEVER forget...
because my doctor told me that I have cancer.

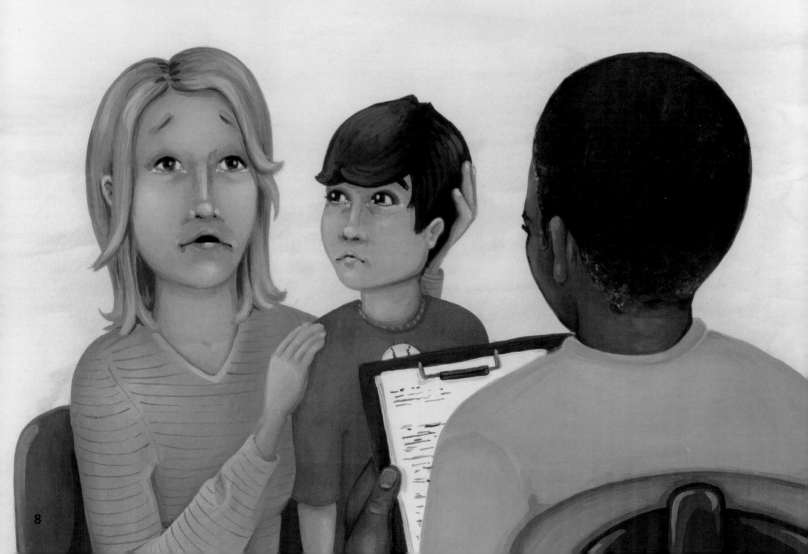

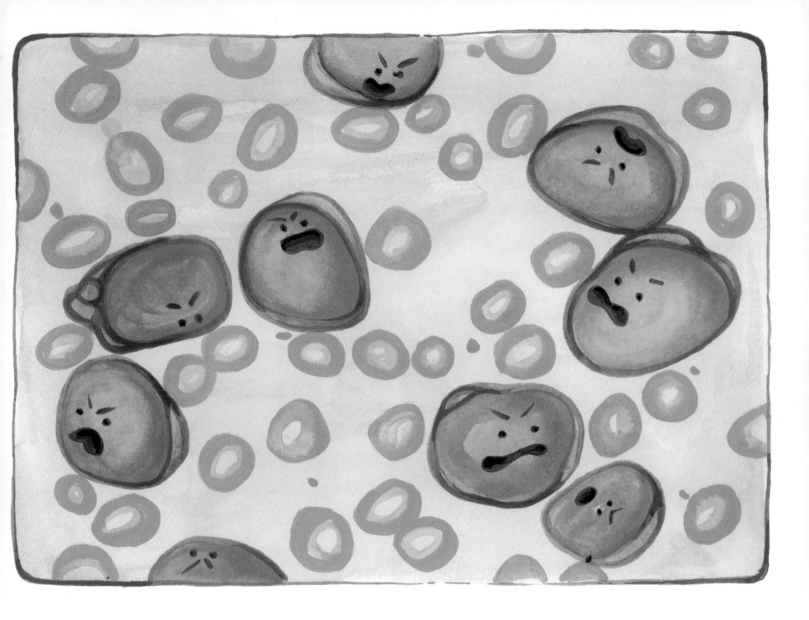

Cancer is a disease that makes some of the cells in your body turn bad and unhealthy. These bad cells grow so fast there isn't enough room for the good cells that are healthy.

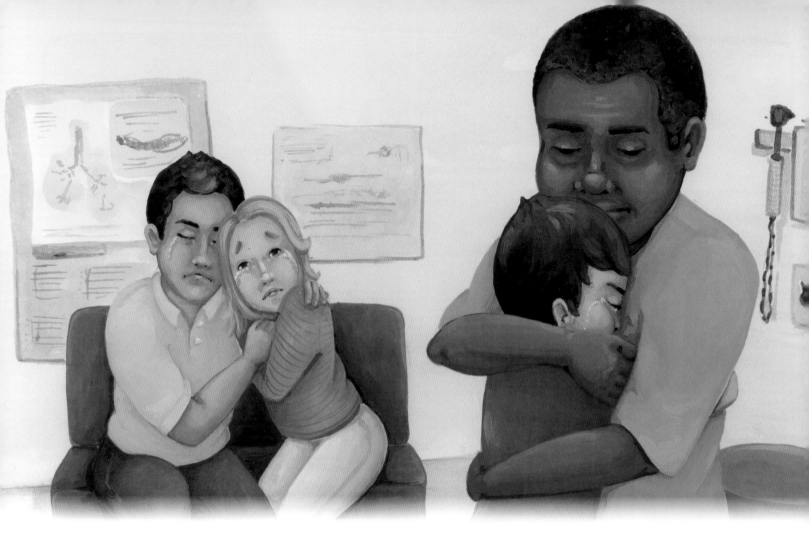

When my doctor first told me that I have cancer, my parents cried, and their eyes looked worried.

I didn't know what to think or how to feel.

Then, my doctor gave me a hug and said:

*"There is a "**CAN**" in cancer.*

*So when your life seems kinda rough,
breathe in and out and clear your head.*

Then think about better stuff."

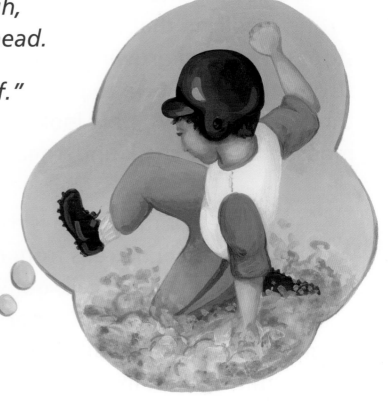

So that's what I did.

I thought about baseball,
and that made me smile.

I went into the hospital right after that and started getting chemo. Chemo is really strong medicine that kills the bad cells and stops them from growing. Chemo is so strong that they have to put it into your body through a port. My port looked like a little mouse that was stuck underneath my skin.

The problem with chemo is that sometimes, it can't tell my bad cells from my good ones, so some of my good cells get wiped out too. This made me feel super yucky inside and out. I felt tired all of the time, and sometimes, I felt like I had the flu.

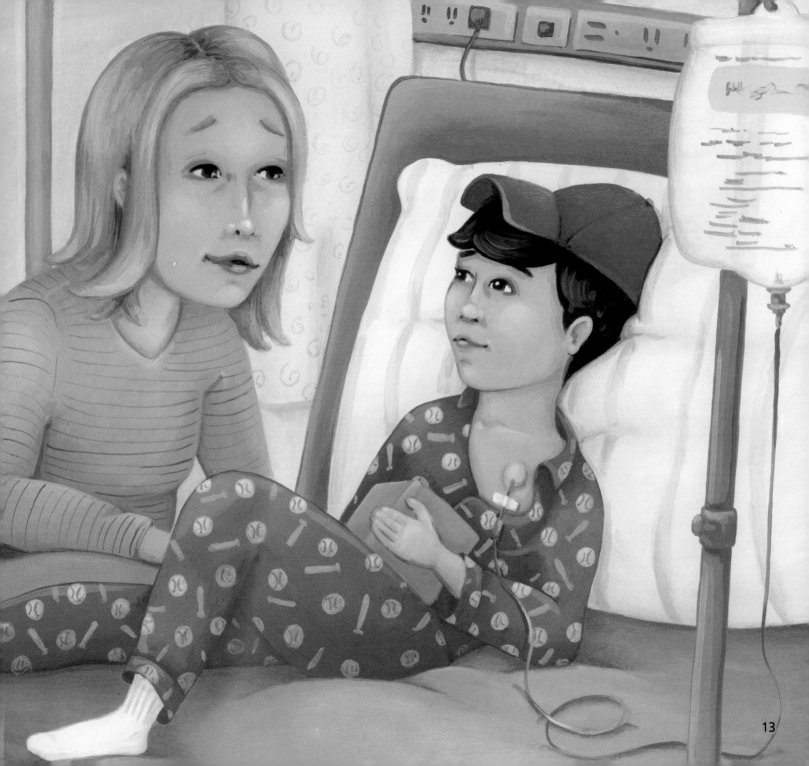

I tried to eat, but even cheese pizza tasted yucky.

Chemo made me really, really sick and that made my parents really, really sad.

One good thing about chemo though, is that the yucky days don't last forever.

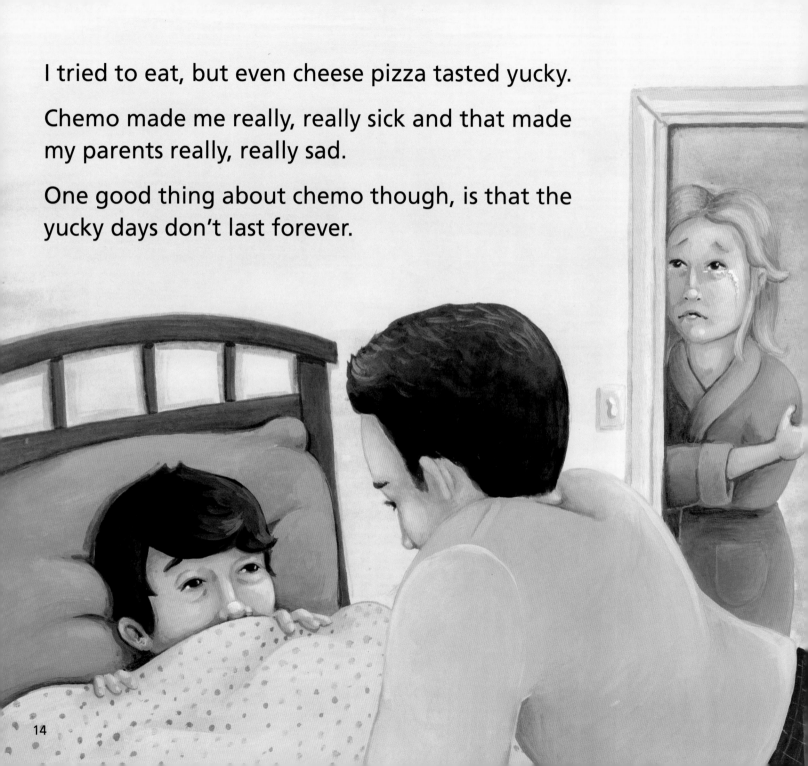

One day, when I was getting my chemo, my mom started to cry and she just couldn't stop.

So I gave her a hug, and then I told her what my doctor told me:

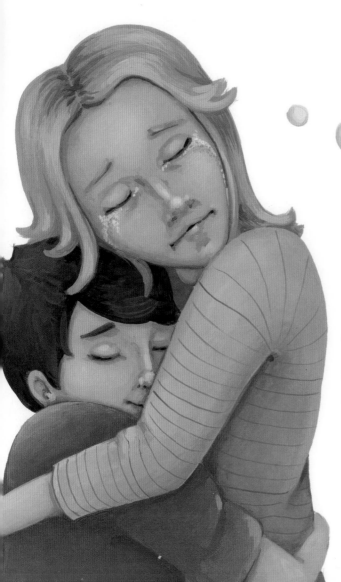

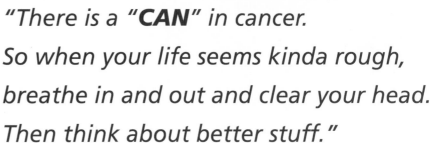

"There is a **"CAN"** *in cancer.*
So when your life seems kinda rough,
breathe in and out and clear your head.
Then think about better stuff."

So that's what my mom did. She thought about the day I was born, and that made her smile.

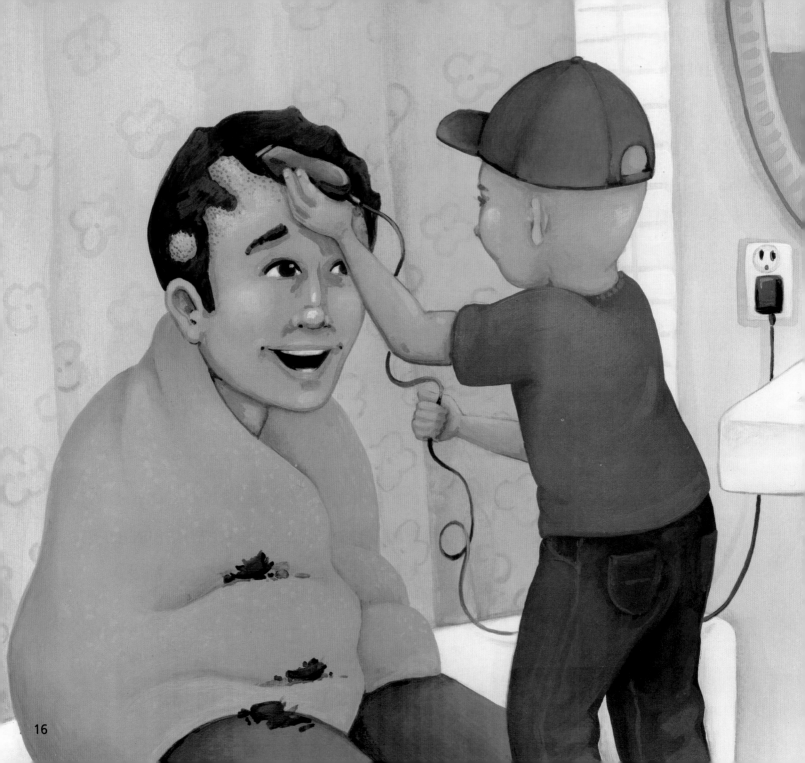

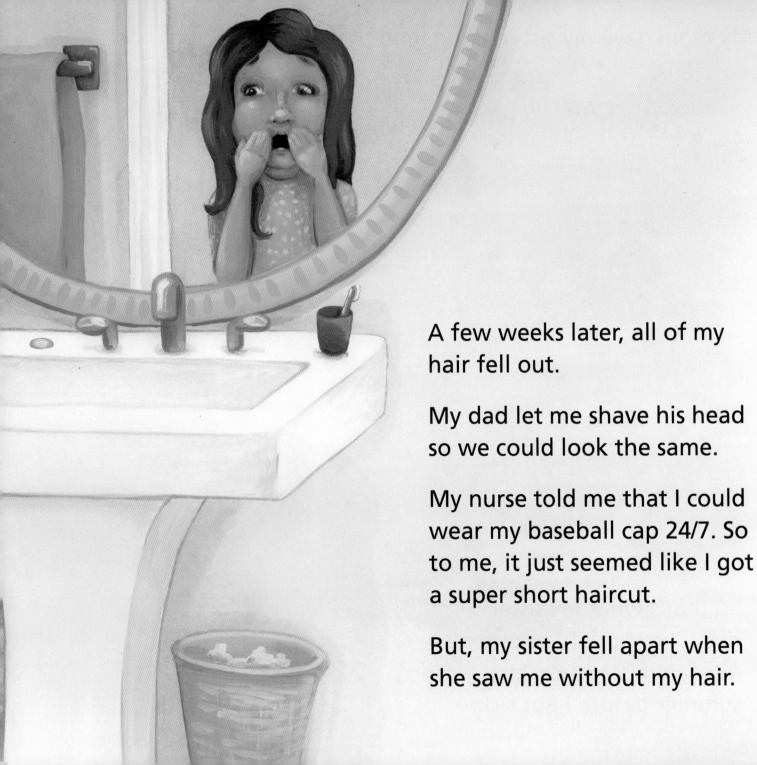

A few weeks later, all of my hair fell out.

My dad let me shave his head so we could look the same.

My nurse told me that I could wear my baseball cap 24/7. So to me, it just seemed like I got a super short haircut.

But, my sister fell apart when she saw me without my hair.

My mom gave my sister a hug, and then she said:

"There is a **"CAN"** in cancer. So when your life seems kinda rough, breathe in and out and clear your head. Then think about better stuff."

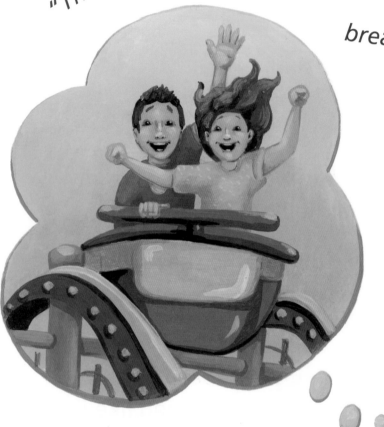

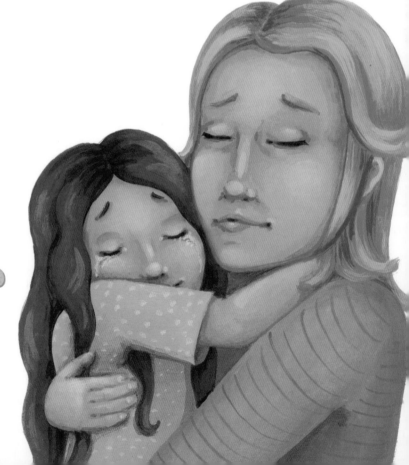

So that's what my sister did. She thought about our family vacation last summer before I got sick.

Then, I let her draw a picture on my bald head
(with washable markers, of course),

and that made her smile.

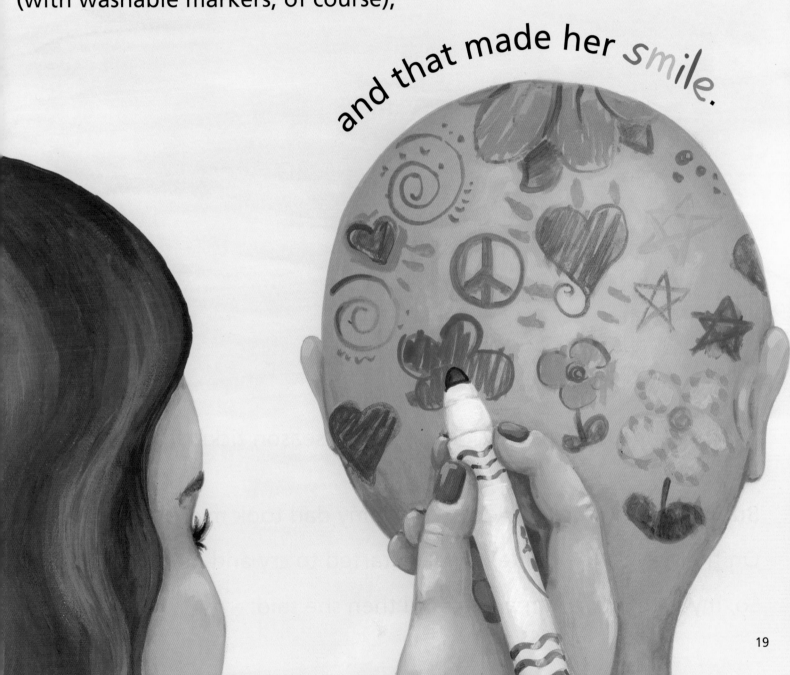

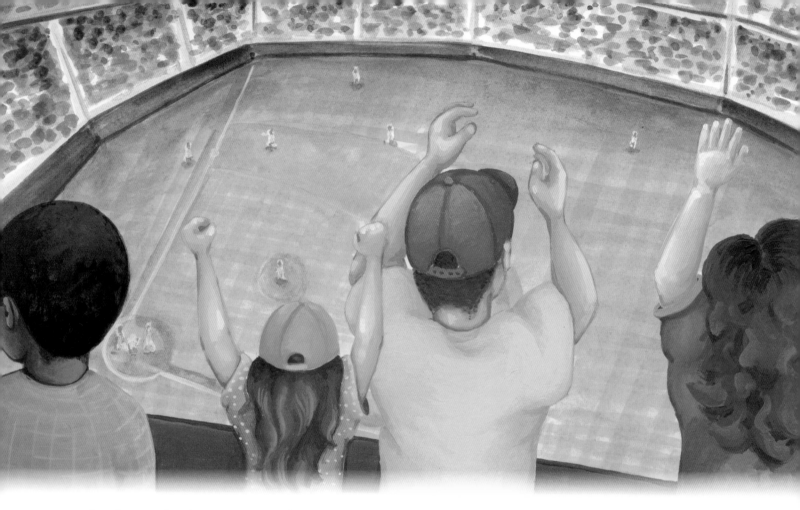

My dad and I have professional baseball season tickets, and we never miss a game!

But last year, I was too sick to go, so my dad took my sister instead.

On the way to the game, my dad started to cry and he couldn't stop.

So, my sister gave him a hug, and then she said:

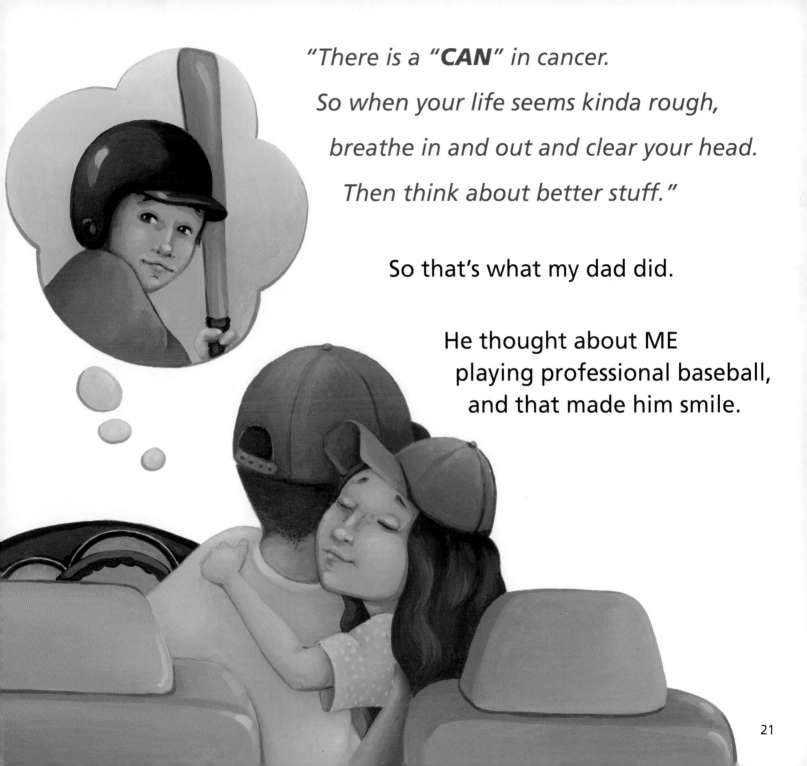

"There is a **"CAN"** in cancer.

So when your life seems kinda rough,

breathe in and out and clear your head.

Then think about better stuff."

So that's what my dad did.

He thought about ME
playing professional baseball,
and that made him smile.

About a week later, my parents and the hospital Child Life Specialist went to my school and talked to my teacher and Nurse Twyla, our school nurse.

The Child Life Specialist told them all about me and about my cancer.

She told them when I would be able to come back to school and when I would need to stay at home.

My parents asked Nurse Twyla to call and let them know when other kids at school were sick. Since chemo kills my good cells too, I can't be around anyone who is sick because their sick germs could make me really, REALLY sick.

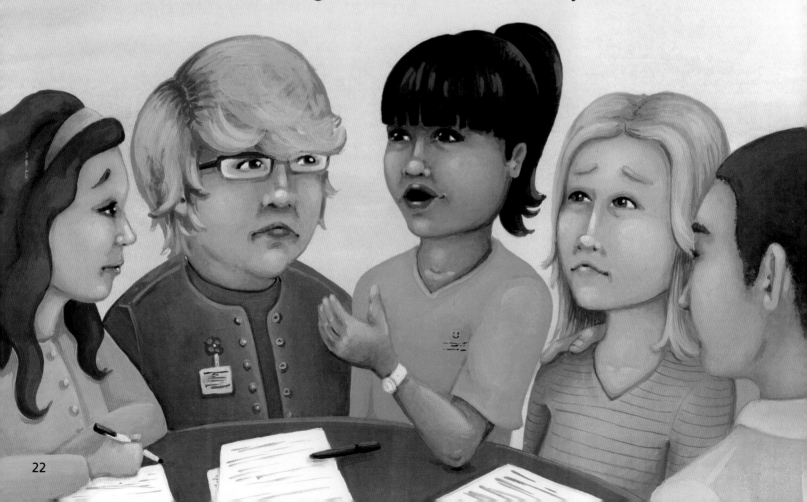

Nurse Twyla and my teacher started to cry. So my dad hugged both of them and said:

*"There is a "**CAN**" in cancer.*

So when your life seems kinda rough,

breathe in and out and clear your head.

Then think about better stuff."

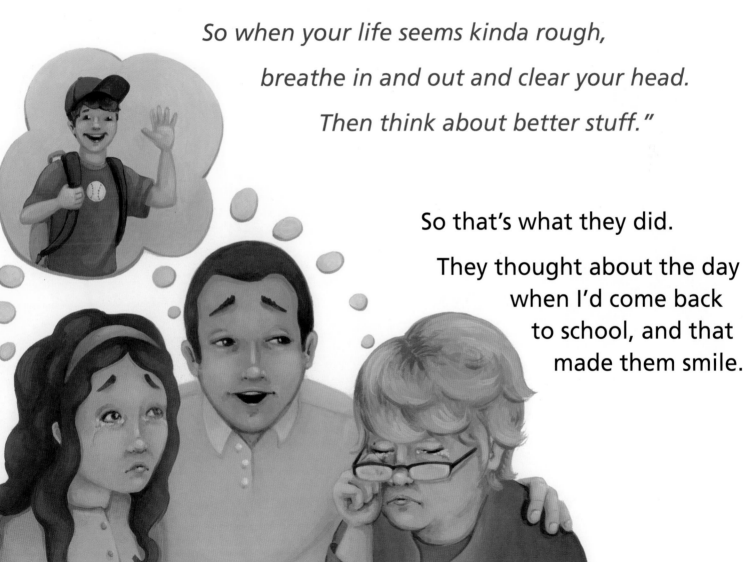

So that's what they did.

They thought about the day when I'd come back to school, and that made them smile.

The next day, my teacher and Nurse Twyla talked to all the kids in my class about me and my cancer.

"Keep sending Eli notes and letters, so he knows what's going on.
He misses every one of you, and he's trying hard to get strong.

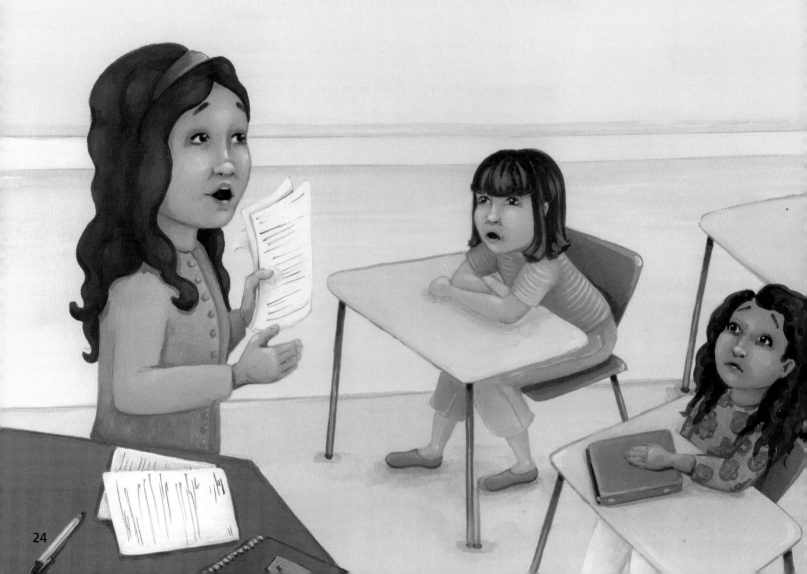

If you go to the hospital to see Eli, call first before you go.
    If Eli doesn't feel that great, they might have to tell you, "NO."

When Eli comes back to school again just treat him like a regular kid.
    He might look and act a bit differently, but treat Eli just like you did."

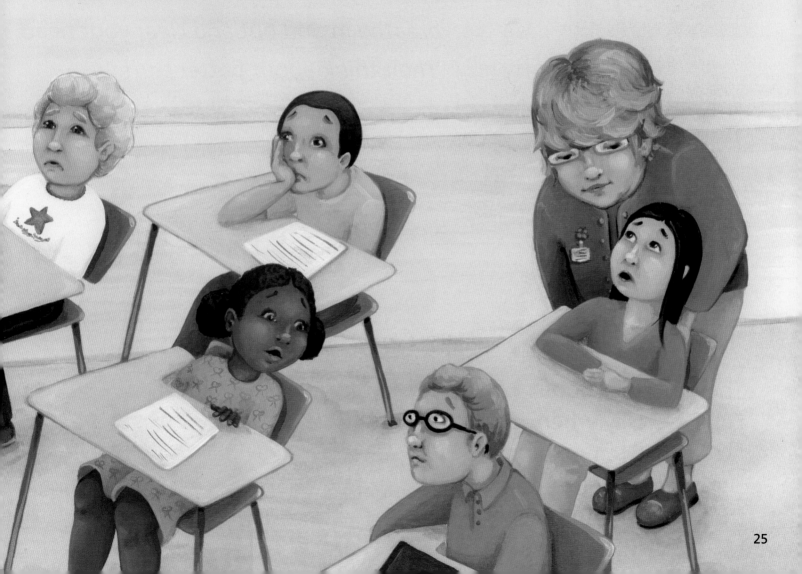

Then, some of the kids in my class started to cry. So my teacher gave them a hug, and then she said:

*"There is a "**CAN**" in cancer.*
So when your life seems kinda rough,
breathe in and out and clear your head.
Then think about better stuff."

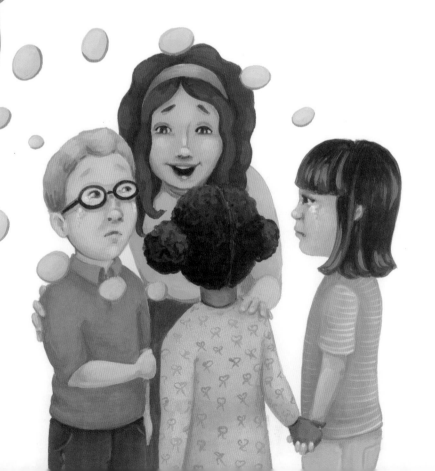

So that's what they did.

They thought about Fall Field Day when I won the Home Run Derby for my class...and that made them smile.

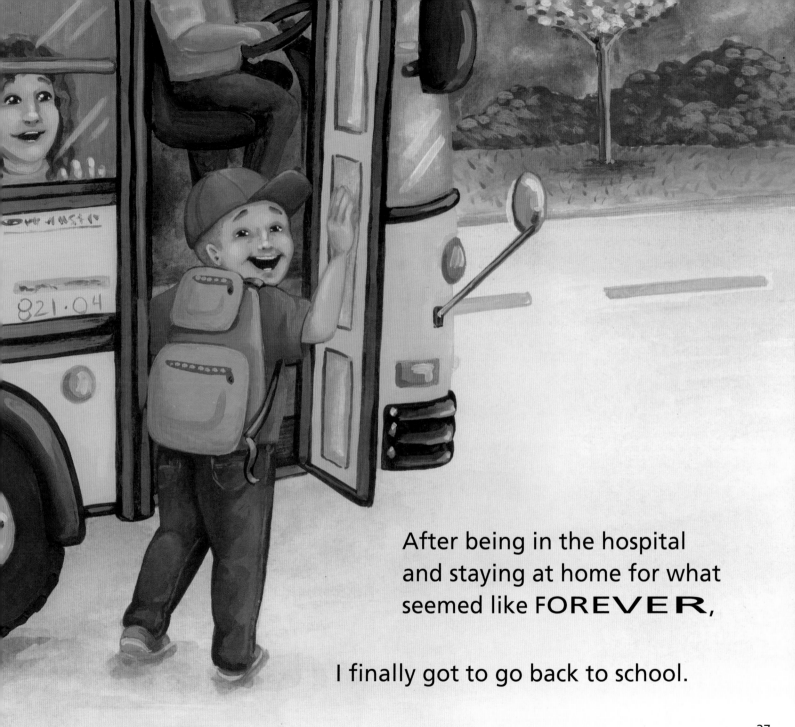

After being in the hospital and staying at home for what seemed like **FOREVER**,

I finally got to go back to school.

My day started out great! But at recess, I struck out both times when I got up to bat, and my team lost...because of me.

I started to cry, and I tried to hide it, but my best friend Ben saw my eyes.

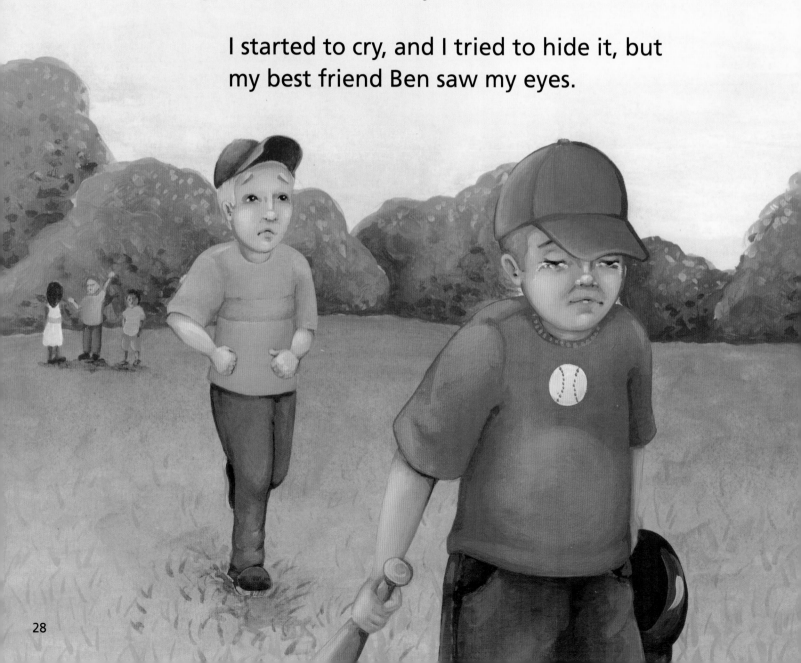

He hugged me, and then he said:

"There is a "CAN" in cancer. So when your life seems kinda rough, breathe in and out and clear your head. Then think about better stuff."

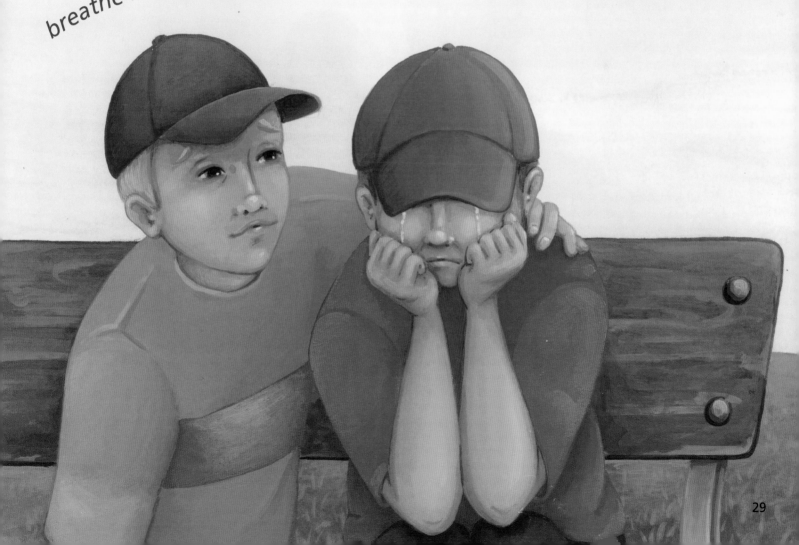

So that's what I did. I thought about me,
and how lucky I am to be here…

And that made me **smile!**

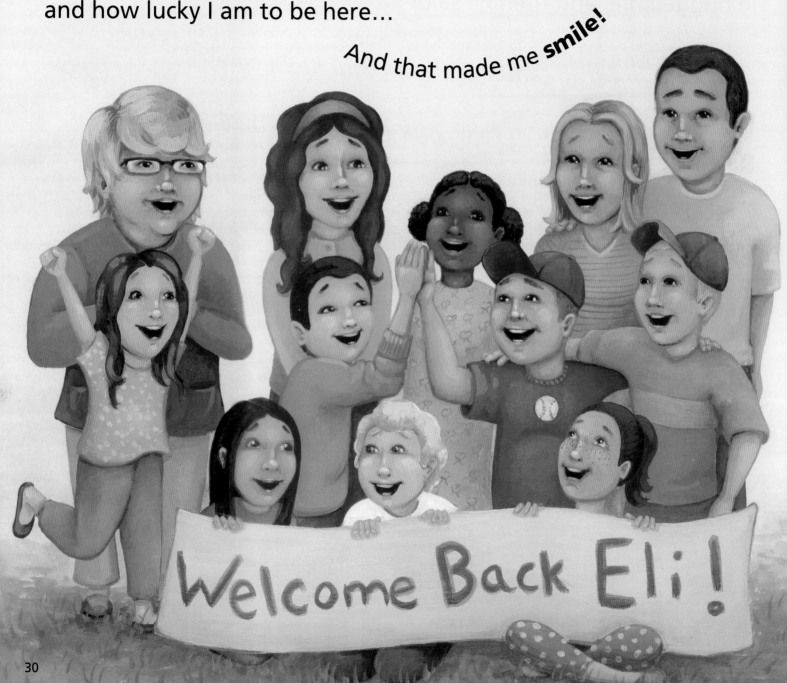

FOR PARENTS:

- Ask questions! From medical terms to a hospital stay or a clinic visit, you will encounter many new situations, and information is KEY!
- You are your child's expert! You know your child better than anyone, making you a crucial member of your child's care team. Talk to the doctors, nurses, and other health care professionals. Your information is vital!
- Benefit from our experience. Social workers and child life specialists are here for you. They can assist you in identifying resources and sharing information in a way your child can understand.
- Try to remain positive in front of your child. Remember…you are your child's coping instructor. His/her attitude will reflect your own.
- Find a private place for conversation, when needed.
- Take a break and try to find quiet time for yourself. You need to remember to take care of yourself so you can stay strong for your child.
- Continue to "parent" your child. Refrain from overindulging or consistently reinforcing bad behaviors that could be difficult to break when your child is healthy again. The goal is to heal your child…not create a behavior monster.
- Be open to accepting offers of help.
- Establish a communication channel to keep family and friends informed. Free website services like CaringBridge or CarePages are designed for medical updates.
- Designate a friend or loved one to provide information updates to others. Save your energy for your child and your family.
- Think about the information you feel comfortable sharing. It's okay to keep some things private.
- Accept that everyone deals with things in their own way. Coping is a unique strategy for all.
- Share household duties and sibling care needs with a spouse, loved ones or friends. Try to stay balanced and remember you can't be everything to everyone all of the time.
- Meet and talk with other families coping with cancer. Find out if your hospital has a support group that you can become a part of.

FOR SIBLINGS:

A cancer diagnosis impacts the entire family. Siblings of all ages share this impact and can experience a wide range of emotions and reactions.

- Introduce siblings to your child's medical team.
- Keep communication open and honest. Children of different ages may need one-on-one conversations with a parent to hear information in a way that they can understand.
- Remain calm and reassuring – create an environment where children will feel comfortable asking questions.
- Always answer your child's questions truthfully with simple answers. You don't need to go into more detail than necessary. Lying to your children or making up facts will ultimately confuse them and could cause them to distrust you in the future.
- You may be asked to repeat your answers several times. Be consistent in your reply, and realize that your repetitive answers are reassuring your child's "need to know" and building upon their sense of security.
- Children often feel out of control when a family illness occurs. Keeping with a familiar routine is very important when trying to reestablish the security of feeling in control.
- Understand that children may feel guilty about a sibling's cancer. They may be fearful of becoming ill themselves or become overly anxious.
- If your child asks a question that you do not know the answer to, it's okay to say, "I don't know."
- Acknowledge and normalize your child's thoughts feelings and reactions. Help children understand why they feel this way.
- Make time for one-on-one outings or moments at home.

- Encourage extended family to reach out to siblings, making them feel special.
- Notify siblings' school, teachers and coaches of family situation.
- Look for support groups, camps or other programs where siblings can connect with peers in similar situations.
- Expect some acting out and/or changes in behavior.
- Reassure your children that many people out there are helping their sibling. Find special ways to involve each sibling so they can feel included in the team.
- Promote positive coping and problem solving skills. Remember – you are your child's coping instructor. Your children are very interested in how you respond. They also may be listening to every word you say when you discuss these events with other adults.
- Emphasize children's resiliency. Fortunately, most children, even those who are exposed to serious illnesses, are quite resilient.

TO EXTENDED FAMILY AND FRIENDS:

There are many ways that you can help us through this time of adjustment. Here are guidelines to help you know what helps and what doesn't:

We need. . .
- To feel that we're not alone.
- Your encouragement.
- Your acknowledgement of what's going on.
- You to listen to us. Listen completely and well. Help us tell the story.
- A break from the hospital for 20 minutes, or to talk as a couple.
- Our child's siblings to feel included.
- You to call before you visit.
- You to understand if we are not up for visitors on a particular day, if we forget to return calls or give updates.
- You to be specific in your offers of help (i.e. delivering meals or helping with a sibling.) We may be too overwhelmed to process general offers such as, "I'm here if you need me."

Please try not to. . .
- Avoid us because you don't know what to say.
- Promise something and not follow through.
- Call us "superwoman," "superman," or a hero.
- Give unsolicited advice.
- Try to relate.
- Compare our situation to others that are not the same.
- Come to visit if your kids are sick.

Thank you for caring!

Love,

Candlelighters of Omaha

A support group for parents, siblings and children with cancer

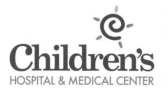

The Hematology/Oncology Program at Children's Hospital & Medical Center in Omaha offers cutting-edge treatment from physicians and staff who understand all aspects of cancer, from the disease process and how best to treat it, to the emotional and social toll that the disease can have not only on the child, but the entire family.

Children's is a member of the Children's Oncology Group (COG), the world's largest, cooperative children's cancer research entity. Doctors and staff at Children's have complete access to the latest research and world-class treatments and are involved in research that helps develop new treatment protocols.

www.ChildrensOmaha.org